ESSENTIAL GUIDE TO SCLERODEMA

Scleroderma Demystified: An Authoritative Guide to Understanding and Managing the Condition

DR. CASEY LOREN

DISCLAIMER

This book's content is only meant to be used for general informative purposes. Although the author has taken great care to ensure the content is accurate and thorough, no warranties or assurances on the information's accuracy, correctness, or reliability are provided. It is recommended that readers employ their own judgment and discretion when applying any material found in this book to their particular situation.

The information in this book is not intended to replace professional advice, nor is the author an expert in any of the subjects covered. It is recommended that readers consult with experienced professionals regarding any particular issues or concerns.

Any name that may be mentioned or referred in this book does not imply endorsement, recommendation, or relationship on the part of the author with any person, entity, good, website, or association. These references are made only for informational purposes and are not meant to be taken as recommendations or endorsements.

The information contained in this book may cause readers to suffer loss or damage, for which the author disclaims all obligation and accountability. The only people accountable for the decisions and actions taken by readers using the information presented are themselves.

Any names, characters, companies, locations, activities, occasions, and incidents referenced in this book are either made up or the result of the author's imagination. Any likeness to real people, living or dead, or to real things is entirely coincidental.

This book's content may change at any time, without prior notice, according to the author. The onus is on the reader to verify whether there have been any updates or revisions.

The reader accepts the conditions of this disclaimer by reading this book. Please do not read this book or use its contents if you do not agree to these terms.

CHAPTER 1

GETTING STARTED WITH SCLERODERMA

The Definitive Resource on Scleroderma

Scleroderma is a skin condition.

Systemic sclerosis, or scleroderma, is an autoimmune rheumatic disease that affects the connective tissues over an extended period. The term "scleroderma" is derived from the Greek words "sclero," meaning hard, and "derma," denoting skin. The disease's most noticeable symptom is a hardening of the skin. Nevertheless, scleroderma has the potential to impact not just the skin but also the internal organs and the vascular system. Scarring and tissue hardening are symptoms of collagen excess, which manifests in the skin and other organs.

Background and Synopsis

In 1836, the Italian physician Carlo Curzio initially introduced the word scleroderma to describe a case of the disease in a young woman. It wasn't until the late 1800s and early 1900s, nevertheless, that comprehensive clinical accounts of the illness began to surface. It is now understood that scleroderma is a multi-symptomatic disorder with several subgroups. It is a subject of continuous research to better understand and treat its varied manifestations since its pathophysiology involves autoimmune, vascular, and fibrotic processes.

The Differences Between Systemic and Localised Scleroderma

There are essentially two primary forms of scleroderma:

Scleroderma that is localized

There are two basic kinds of localized scleroderma, both of which primarily impact the skin:

1. Symptoms of **Morphea** include areas of skin that are hard and discolored. These patches might be small and localized or larger and more dispersed.

2. One kind of scleroderma, known as **linear sclerosis**, causes the skin to thicken in a distinct pattern, most commonly on the forehead, arms, or legs. It has the potential to stunt a child's bone and tissue development.

Systemic sclerosis, also known as scleroderma,

All organs in the body are impacted by systemic scleroderma. Then it is subdivided into:

1. Typically manifests on the extremities (feet, face, and hands) in cases of **Limited Cutaneous Systemic Sclerosis**. Although it often advances more slowly than the diffuse form, it can

potentially affect internal organs. Included in this category is the subtype known as CREST syndrome, which stands for calcinosis, Raynaud's phenomenon, esophageal dysfunction, sclerodactyly, and telangiectasia.

2. **Diffuse Cutaneous Systemic Sclerosis**: This condition causes the skin all over the body, including the trunk, to thicken. It progresses quickly and can eventually impact internal organs like the lungs, heart, kidneys, and gastrointestinal tract.

Demographics and Prevalence

About 2.5 million people across the globe are affected by the rare disease scleroderma. The female-to-male ratio is approximately 4:1, meaning that it is more prevalent in women. It usually starts between thirty and fifty years old, but it can happen at any age. There is an increased incidence and potential for more severe symptoms among certain racial and ethnic groups.

Typical Indications and Outcomes

Scleroderma symptoms can range from mild to severe, depending on the kind and organs affected. However, some of the most prevalent indicators include:

- **Skin Changes**: The skin becomes thicker and harder, especially on the face, hands, and fingers.

The **Raynaud's Phenomenon** is a medical disorder in which exposure to cold or stress causes the fingers and toes to turn white or blue.

As a result of inflammation and skin tightening, you may have joint pain and stiffness.

Acid reflux, trouble swallowing, and gastrointestinal problems are all examples of **Digestive Problems**.

- **Respiratory Problems**: Lung involvement causes dry coughing and shortness of breath.

- **Diseases of the Kidneys**: May cause high blood pressure and kidney failure.

- **Dealing With the Heart**: This includes, in extreme circumstances, arrhythmias and heart failure.

Causes and Factors That Pose a Risk

While researchers have yet to pinpoint a single cause for scleroderma, they do believe that environmental, immune system, and genetic variables all have a role. Potential dangers encompass:

- **Hereditary Predisposition**: Autoimmune illnesses run in families.

Chemical and solvent exposure, as well as viral infections, are examples of **Environmental Triggers**.

- Inflammation and fibrosis can result from **immune system dysfunction**, which is defined as abnormal immunological responses.

Initial Steps in Diagnosing Scleroderma

Clinical assessment, laboratory testing, and imaging studies are the usual components of a diagnosis:

- The clinical examination involves looking for changes in the skin, symptoms of Raynaud's phenomenon, and other physical indicators.

To detect specific autoantibodies, including anti-centromere and anti-Scl-70, a blood test can be performed.

- **Imaging**: Methods for assessing the involvement of internal organs by imaging, such as echocardiograms, pulmonary function tests, and gastrointestinal examinations.

In rare cases, a skin biopsy may be necessary to confirm the diagnosis.

How Scleroderma Affects Regular Life

Daily activities and quality of life can be greatly impacted by living with scleroderma:

Stiffness in the joints and changes to the skin can limit mobility and dexterity.

The body's constant fight against inflammation and fibrosis is a typical cause of chronic exhaustion, which manifests as fatigue.

- **Digestive Issues**: Medications and changes to one's diet may be necessary to alleviate symptoms.

- **Respiratory Issues**: Lessened capacity for lung function might restrict physical exertion.

Adjustments may be required to accommodate physical constraints and medical appointments, which can impact both work and social life.

The Mental and Emotional Elements

Psychological difficulties, such as: due to the chronic and unpredictable character of scleroderma

- **Depression and Anxiety**: As a result of the physical restrictions, ongoing discomfort, and effects on one's physical appearance.

Problems with one's body image can have an impact on one's sense of self-worth and one's ability to interact socially.

- **Stress Management**: It may be very important to learn coping mechanisms and to seek help from mental health experts.

Treatment Approaches: A Comprehensive Review

Treatments for scleroderma focus on symptom management, problem prevention, and quality of life improvement; nevertheless, a solution is not yet available.

Immunosuppressants, corticosteroids, and other medications are used to address some symptoms, such as Raynaud's phenomenon and gastrointestinal difficulties.

- **Physical Therapy**: To preserve mobility and control discomfort.

Assisting with routine tasks and making necessary adjustments is the goal of occupational therapy.

Changes to one's way of life, include giving up smoking, eating healthier, and making exercise a regular part of one's routine.

To keep an eye on how your organs are doing and make any required adjustments to your treatment, it is important to have regular checkups with a multidisciplinary team.

To sum up, scleroderma is an intricate and diverse illness that calls for an all-encompassing strategy for diagnosis, therapy, and management.

Together, patients, carers, and healthcare practitioners can better understand this complex disorder and its many facets to better assist those living with it and improve their quality of life.

CHAPTER 2

EXPLORING THE DIFFERENT FORMS OF SCLERODERMA

Morphea: Localised Scleroderma

One form of localized scleroderma, known as morphea, mostly manifests as skin lesions. Hardened, discolored patches of skin can manifest in various sizes, from localized spots to bigger, more extensive areas. A reddish or dark border typically surrounds a white or purple center in these patches. Rarely, morphea can induce localized muscle weakness or stiffness, however, it usually doesn't impact internal organs. It is thought that an aberrant immune reaction causes inflammation and excessive collagen formation in the skin, which is the exact etiology of Morphea, however, no one knows for sure.

The Linear Scleroderma and Localised Scleroderma

Another kind of localized scleroderma, linear scleroderma usually shows up as a band or streak of rigid skin. Although this scleroderma type can manifest on other parts of the body, most commonly the limbs (especially the arms and legs), it can also manifest on the scalp and face. Some symptoms of linear scleroderma include localized skin tightening, stiffness of the joints, and weakening of the muscles in the affected area. Sometimes it spreads to the deeper layers of tissue, interfering with things like bones and joints. It is believed that immune system malfunction and aberrant collagen formation are the exact causes of linear scleroderma, similar to Morphea. However, the specific cause is still not entirely understood.

Limited Cutaneous Expansion in Systemic Scleroderma

Skin, blood vessels, and specific internal organs like the esophagus are the main targets of limited cutaneous systemic scleroderma, which is also called limited scleroderma or CREST syndrome (Calcinosis, Raynaud's phenomenon, Esophageal dysmotility, Sclerodactyly, Telangiectasia). The condition typically begins with Raynaud's phenomenon, in which the finger and toe blood vessels contract in reaction to cold or stress, resulting in painful color changes and tingling. Sclerodactyly, telangiectasia, thickening skin on the hands, cheeks, and feet, difficulty swallowing, and calcinosis, which are calcium deposits under the skin, are other possible symptoms. Telangiectasia is characterized by tiny dilated blood vessels near the skin's surface. Esophageal involvement can make swallowing difficult. In contrast to diffuse cutaneous systemic sclerosis, which can spread rapidly, limited cutaneous systemic sclerosis often develops more subtly and affects fewer organs.

Diffuse Cutaneous Systemic Scleroderma

The skin and internal organs like the lungs, heart, kidneys, and gastrointestinal tract are both impacted by diffuse cutaneous systemic sclerosis, a more severe and fast-advancing type of systemic sclerosis. A thickening of the skin across a substantial portion of the body, sometimes affecting the face, arms, legs, and trunk, is a hallmark of this condition. Pulmonary hypertension, interstitial lung disease, renal failure, and cardiac issues are among the serious consequences that may develop from diffuse scleroderma. Aggressive symptom control and the use of immunosuppressive drugs to decrease inflammation and halt disease progression are common components of treatment for diffuse cutaneous systemic sclerosis.

A Distinct Subset of Scleroderma: Sine Scleroderma

Internal organ involvement without noticeable skin changes is seen in rare cases of sine scleroderma, a subtype of systemic scleroderma. The lack of skin thickening, a hallmark of other types of scleroderma, makes this condition difficult to identify. When other organs aren't working properly, patients may experience symptoms including trouble breathing (from the lungs), heart palpitations or chest discomfort (from the heart), gastrointestinal issues, or renal failure. A multidisciplinary strategy combining experts in rheumatology, pulmonology, cardiology, and other related specialties is typically necessary for the careful monitoring and therapy of organ problems in patients with sinus scleroderma.

Diseases Affecting Mixed Connective Tissues and Overlap Syndromes

Scleroderma, lupus, rheumatoid arthritis, polymyositis, and other autoimmune diseases can coexist in a single person, a phenomenon known as overlap syndrome or mixed connective tissue disease (MCTD). A variety of symptoms, including aches and pains in the joints, changes in the skin, weakened muscles, and even involvement of internal organs, can indicate the presence of these disorders. To manage the unique symptoms and problems of overlap syndromes and MCTD, thorough evaluations and treatments are required.

Special Considerations for Children with Scleroderma

Although uncommon in children, scleroderma can nonetheless strike this age range. Skin involvement, joint complaints, and internal organ issues can manifest differently in children with scleroderma compared to adults. Medical professionals who are well-versed in the specific difficulties of treating scleroderma in children, such as pediatric rheumatologists, are essential to the treatment of this illness in children. Prolonged monitoring of organ function, anti-inflammatory medicine, and physical therapy to keep joints mobile may all be part of the treatment plan.

Discover Rare Scleroderma Varieties

Above, we covered the most common varieties of scleroderma. However, many unusual variants and subtypes of the disease can cause different symptoms and difficulties. Scleroderma sine scleroderma is a variation that involves internal organs without major skin changes; eosinophilic fasciitis mostly impacts the deep connective tissues and can induce intense muscle and joint pain. Thorough evaluation and tailored treatment strategies are necessary for other uncommon types of scleroderma, which can affect certain organ systems or display unusual symptoms.

A Comparison of Systemic Scleroderma with Localised Scleroderma

Morphea and linear scleroderma are forms of localized scleroderma that cause thicker and more rigid skin in specific locations by affecting the skin and underlying tissues. The prognosis is better for these types of scleroderma than for systemic scleroderma because they usually do not affect internal organs. However, systemic scleroderma can impact several organ systems, such as the skin, arteries, lungs, heart, kidneys, and digestive system. It necessitates all-encompassing care to treat the skin and internal organs because of the increased risk of consequences.

How Scleroderma Develops and Progresses

The type and severity of scleroderma determine how the disease develops and at what stage it is staged. Typically, localized scleroderma moves at a snail's pace and can get better or stay the same with time and treatment. Organ damage and problems can occur more quickly in systemic scleroderma, especially in the diffuse cutaneous form. To make treatment options and track the evolution of scleroderma, it is necessary to stage the disease by evaluating the level of skin involvement, organ function, and overall severity. When it comes to controlling scleroderma and making necessary adjustments to treatment, nothing is more important than regular follow-up examinations, symptom monitoring, laboratory testing, and imaging investigations.

CHAPTER 3

ISSUES AND SIDE EFFECTS

Alterations to the Skin and Hardening

Skin alterations, such as thickening, hardness, and tightening, are characteristic of scleroderma. Reduced mobility and flexibility may result in issues with the hands, face, and other parts of the body. Shininess, tightness, and the appearance of hyper- or hypopigmented patches are all possible side effects of this treatment. Proper skincare can help avoid dryness and cracking, while therapies such as topical ointments or phototherapy can alleviate symptoms.

Raynaud's Illusion

Scleroderma frequently manifests as Raynaud's Phenomenon, a condition in which the blood vessels constrict in reaction to cold or stress, resulting in diminished blood circulation to the extremities. Colour changes (from white to blue to red), tingling, numbness, and pain can all be caused by this. Keep the limbs warm, stay away from things that cause it, take medicine to increase blood flow, and in extreme cases, surgery may be necessary for management.

Digestive Problems

Symptoms of scleroderma that impact the gastrointestinal tract include heartburn, dysphagia, gas, diarrhea, constipation, and bloating. This occurs because the digestive system makes use of smooth muscles. In cases of serious problems, such as strictures, surgical procedures may be necessary in addition to dietary changes and symptom management drugs.

Fibrosis and Hypertension as Pulmonary Complications

Scleroderma can cause pulmonary problems such as pulmonary arterial hypertension (PAH) and interstitial lung disease (fibrosis). Reduced lung function and difficulty breathing are symptoms of fibrosis, which is characterized by scarring of the lung tissue. The heart might be burdened by the elevated blood pressure in the lungs caused by PAH. Regular monitoring, symptom and progression-management medicines, oxygen therapy, and, in extreme circumstances, lung transplantation are all part of the management plan.

The Role of the Renal System and Emergencies

Damage to the kidneys, brought on by scleroderma, impairs their capacity to filter waste and control fluid levels. Serious consequences such as kidney failure and abruptly rising blood pressure are hallmarks of scleroderma renal crisis, which can develop from this. Dialysis or kidney transplantation may be necessary in extreme cases, in addition to medication to preserve the kidneys, controlling blood pressure, and close monitoring of kidney function as part of management.

The Musculoskeletal System

Joint discomfort, stiffness, inflammation, and weakening of the muscles are all symptoms of scleroderma's musculoskeletal complications. Mobility and daily activities can be impacted by these symptoms. Treatment includes physiotherapy, exercise regimens, anti-inflammatory and pain drugs, and behavioral changes to enhance mobility and well-being.

Hypertension and Other Heart Problems

Problems such as arrhythmias, pericarditis, myocardial fibrosis, and heart failure can develop when scleroderma impacts the cardiovascular system. Management may include regular heart monitoring, medication to alleviate symptoms and avoid complications, changes in lifestyle (such as giving up smoking and eating healthier), and occasionally surgical procedures.

Problems with the Mouth and Teeth

Scleroderma can cause a variety of oral and dental problems, such as xerostomia (dry mouth), trismus (difficulty opening the mouth), gum disease, and tooth decay. The best way to deal with these problems is to see a dentist regularly, practice good oral hygiene, use saliva substitutes as needed, and treat any specific oral troubles that may arise.

Tiredness and Overall Health

Scleroderma symptoms, including fatigue, can be very disabling. Possible causes include the disease's general effect on one's physical and mental health, as well as specific symptoms like pain and insomnia. Pacing oneself, making a list of to-dos, getting enough sleep, managing stress, and, in certain cases, medication or counseling can all help with managing fatigue.

Identifying and Handling Excessive Reactions

When scleroderma flares up, symptoms including skin changes, discomfort, exhaustion, or organ involvement can get worse. Understanding what sets off flare-ups and how to spot them early is crucial. Reducing the severity of flare-ups and preventing consequences requires management strategies such as regular check-ins with healthcare practitioners, course corrections as needed, behavioral changes, and self-care.

In the context of scleroderma management, these concerns are all interrelated, which emphasizes the need for a multidisciplinary approach that includes dermatologists, pulmonologists, nephrologists, rheumatologists, and gastroenterologists, among others, to offer thorough care. To improve outcomes and quality of life for people with scleroderma, it is crucial to check their condition often, intervene when necessary, and educate patients.

CHAPTER 4
EVALUATION AND EVALUATION

Medical Evaluation

To begin the process of diagnosing scleroderma, a comprehensive physical examination, review of the patient's medical history, and assessment of any symptoms are all part of the initial clinical examination. Thickened skin, Raynaud's phenomenon, and telangiectasias are some of the telltale indications that doctors look for. In addition, they might check for gastrointestinal problems, muscular weakness, and joint pain. Additional diagnostic testing will be guided by the comprehensive information gathered.

The Importance of Autoantibody Testing

Crucial in the diagnosis of scleroderma, autoantibody tests aid in the identification of certain antibodies linked to the condition. Some examples of autoantibodies are:

• Antinuclear antibodies (ANA): This is a common finding in individuals with scleroderma.

Anti-Scl-70, also known as anti-topoisomerase I, is associated with systemic sclerosis of the skin.

Limited cutaneous systemic sclerosis is linked to **anti-centromere antibodies (ACA)**.

- An increased incidence of renal crisis is associated with diffuse skin involvement and **Anti-RNA Polymerase III**.

These diagnostic procedures aid in the subtyping of scleroderma and the prediction of its possible consequences, as well as in differentiating it from other autoimmune illnesses.

Pictures from Imaging Exams: X-rays, CT Scan, and MRI

To determine the extent of involvement and potential consequences in the internal organs of scleroderma patients, imaging investigations are crucial:

Radiographs: **X-rays:** These can reveal pulmonary fibrosis, joint degeneration, and calcinosis.

- Computed tomography scans: These images show the lungs in great detail and can be used to diagnose pulmonary fibrosis and interstitial lung disease.

High-resolution images of soft tissues are provided by magnetic resonance imaging (MRI). These images can be used to assess inflammation in muscles and joints, identify early-stage involvement of internal organs, and more.

These imaging methods are useful for tracking the development of a disease and determining its extent.

Evaluation of Pulmonary Function

Critical for the detection and monitoring of lung involvement in scleroderma, pulmonary function tests (PFTs) evaluate lung function. Important PFTs cover:

One way to diagnose restrictive lung disease is via a spirometry test, which measures the amount of air that is inhaled and exhaled.

- **DLCO:** Measures the lungs' ability to diffuse carbon monoxide gas from the air to the blood, which is frequently diminished in interstitial lung disease.

Evaluate the overall lung capacity as well as the functional residual capacity (Lung Volumes).

The development of lung disease can be monitored and treatment choices made with the use of regular PFTs.

Heart Monitoring and Echocardiograms

A non-invasive diagnostic tool, echocardiograms use ultrasound to produce pictures of the heart. When it comes to finding:

Pressure buildup in the pulmonary arteries, also known as pulmonary arterial hypertension (PAH), is a common complication of scleroderma.

"Pericardial effusion" refers to the buildup of fluid surrounding the heart.

- **Cardiac Dysfunction:** Evaluating the efficiency of the heart's muscles and valves.

Arrhythmias and other cardiac irregularities can be detected by Holter monitoring and other methods of heart monitoring.

The When and Why of Skin Biopsies

A little piece of skin tissue is removed for examination in a lab, a process known as a biopsy. Usually, they are carried out when:

- A histological confirmation is necessary to resolve the uncertainty around the diagnosis.

- To identify scleroderma as distinct from other skin diseases.

- To see how bad the inflammation and fibrosis are on the skin.

Scleroderma can be confirmed and the extent of skin involvement can be learned from biopsy results.

Examining Nailfold Capillaries with Capillaroscopy

Examining the capillaries at the base of the fingernails is possible with capillaroscopy, a non-invasive procedure. Scleroderma can be better diagnosed with its help because it shows:

- **Capillary Patterns That Aren't Normal:** Examples include swollen or twisted capillaries.

A decrease in the total number of capillaries is known as capillary dropout.

A micro hematoma is a tiny blood clot.

The results of capillaroscopy can confirm the presence of scleroderma and shed light on the extent to which microvascular involvement is present.

Eliminating Other Possible Causes: Differential Diagnosis

Excluding other disorders that present with the same symptoms requires a differential diagnosis. Here are some conditions that can be mistaken for scleroderma:

- SLE, or systemic lupus erythematosus,

- **Arthritis Rheumatoid**

- Dysmyositis (sometimes known as polymyositis)

MCTD stands for "mixed connective tissue disease."

- Morphea, or localized scleroderma

Differentiating scleroderma from these other illnesses requires a thorough clinical evaluation, imaging tests, and autoantibody testing.

Studying Genetics and Testing

Genetic factors play a role in the development of scleroderma, although the condition is not directly inherited. Heredity studies and testing center on:

Find the genetic markers that are linked to a higher risk.

- Comprehending the hereditary origins of different sorts of diseases.

Delving into the interplay between genes and the environment that set off the cancer.

Genetic discoveries that may provide new therapeutic targets and personalized treatment techniques are the focus of ongoing study.

Maintaining Consistent Tracking and Follow-Up

Scleroderma management and complication prevention require regular monitoring and follow-up. That includes:

Evaluating symptoms and physical findings is part of the **routine clinical assessments**.

- **Laboratory Tests:** Tracking levels of autoantibodies and the functioning of organs.

- Using imaging and PFTs, we can monitor the course of diseases and the involvement of organs.

Patient Education: Raising awareness of symptoms that may indicate the worsening of a patient's condition and taking steps to ensure that they comply with their treatment plan.

To maximize therapy efficacy and patient satisfaction, it is essential to conduct follow-up appointments at regular intervals.

Emphasizing the significance of a thorough and interdisciplinary approach, this guide offers a thorough review of the diagnostic and monitoring methods necessary for managing scleroderma.

CHAPTER 4

OPTIONS FOR TREATMENT AND MANAGEMENT

An Overview of Pharmacological Treatments

Medications for scleroderma work to alleviate symptoms, delay the worsening of the illness and enhance overall well-being. Due to the multi-system nature of scleroderma, treatment plans are typically individualized based on the patient's unique set of symptoms.

Agents that weaken the immune system

Scleroderma is characterized by an overactive immune system, which can be alleviated with the help of immunosuppressive medications. Some of the most common immunosuppressants are:

Methotrexate is a common medication for the treatment of skin and joint problems.

When it comes to skin and lung involvement, **mycophenolate mofetil** works well.

Cyclophosphamide is mainly prescribed to patients with advanced lung disease.

In cases where mycophenolate mofetil is not an option, azathioprine is sometimes prescribed instead.

Side effects such as an increased risk of infection, liver toxicity, and bone marrow suppression can occur with these medications, while they can help reduce inflammation and fibrosis.

Treatments that Reverse Fibrosis

The goal of anti-fibrotic treatments is to lessen or eliminate the need for scar tissue (fibrosis). Among the agents that are now under study or in use are:

One such medicine is **nintedanib**, which is a scleroderma-associated anti-fibrotic medication used to treat interstitial lung disease.

One such anti-fibrotic drug being studied for scleroderma lung illness is **Pirfenidone**.

The tyrosine kinase inhibitor imatinib is one of the drugs under investigation for its ability to lessen fibrosis.

Research into these treatments is on the rise, and they aim to tackle the fibrotic processes in scleroderma directly.

The Raynaud's Phenomenon and Vasodilators

Scleroderma frequently manifests as Raynaud's syndrome, in which blood vessels suddenly constrict. Vasodilators are helpful because they increase blood flow by expanding the blood arteries. Here are some options:

First-line treatments frequently include **calcium channel blockers**, such as nifedipine and amlodipine.

In more serious instances, phosphodiesterase inhibitors like sildenafil may be helpful.

Analogues of prostacyclin: iloprost, for example, is prescribed for very severe digital ulcers.

- **Bosentan and other endothelin receptor antagonists**: they are useful for both treating severe instances and preventing the development of new ulcers.

In addition to preventing consequences like digital ulcers, these drugs can greatly lessen the severity and frequency of Raynaud's attacks.

Treating Irritable Bowel Syndromes

The esophagus, stomach, and intestines are all affected by scleroderma, which can cause mild to severe gastrointestinal (GI) involvement. Management methods consist of:

- **Medications that block the reversal of proton pumping, such as omeprazole,** for the treatment of gastroesophageal reflux disease (GERD).

To alleviate gastroparesis symptoms and improve stomach emptying, **prokinetic agents** like metoclopramide are used.

- **Antibiotics**: Used to treat scleroderma-related SIBO (small intestine bacterial overgrowth).

Stool softeners and laxatives: For the treatment of constipation.

Eating smaller, more frequent meals and avoiding foods that cause reflux are examples of dietary alterations that can be tailored to alleviate symptoms.

A mix of pharmaceutical therapies and behavioral modifications is necessary for the effective management of gastrointestinal problems.

Interventions and Treatments for the Pulmonary System

Scleroderma patients should be very concerned about the possibility of pulmonary consequences, especially ILD and PAH. Here are some treatments:

ILD can be helped with immunosuppressive therapy, which includes medications like cyclophosphamide and mycophenolate mofetil.

ILD-targeting **anti-fibrotic drugs**, such as nintedanib.

Medications such as bosentan, sildenafil, and epoprostenol are examples of prostacyclins, PDE inhibitors, and endothelin receptor antagonists used to treat PAH.

For those experiencing severe hypoxemia, **oxygen therapy** may be necessary.

For cases that have not responded to other treatments, lung transplantation may be an option.

The key to better results is finding pulmonary involvement early and treating it.

Occupational and Physical Therapy

Retaining mobility and everyday functioning is greatly aided by physical and occupational therapy. Possible interventions are:

- **Exercises that improve range of motion**: To keep joints flexible and avoid contractures.

- Exercises that build muscle and stamina are known as **strengthening exercises**.

Assistive devices: Things like braces and splints that help with everyday activities and enhance quality of life.

To alleviate pain and maximize comfort, consider **ergonomic modifications** for your house or office.

Individualized exercise and rehabilitation regimens are created in close collaboration between patients and therapists.

Modifying One's Lifestyle and Prioritising Self-Care

Essential components of managing scleroderma include making lifestyle adjustments and practicing self-care. Here are some suggestions:

- To improve circulation and reduce the risk of problems, it is recommended to quit smoking.

- **Healthy eating habits**: To alleviate gastrointestinal issues and promote general wellness.

To keep heart health and muscle strength in good shape, regular exercise is essential.

- **Skincare**: To control dry skin and avoid ulcers.

- **Improved symptom management**: By practicing mindfulness and relaxation techniques, as stress makes symptoms worse.

Collaborative effort between patients and healthcare providers is strongly encouraged.

Non-Conventional and Allied Medical Practices

Additional symptom relief and improved health can be achieved through alternative and complementary therapies. Here are some options:

To alleviate pain and improve blood flow, acupuncture is a viable option.

To alleviate stress and increase range of motion, try massage therapy.

• **Herbal supplements**: Evening primrose oil is one example; nonetheless, it is important to use these with caution and under a doctor's supervision.

Yoga and tai chi are examples of mind-body techniques that can improve physical function and alleviate stress.

These therapies should be used in conjunction with traditional treatments, not in place of them, despite their potential benefits.

Tracking Progress and Modifying Therapy

To properly manage scleroderma, it is essential to assess the condition often and make adjustments to medication as needed. That includes:

- **Regular check-ups**: To track the development of the disease and the efficacy of the treatment.

- **Blood tests**: To judge how well organs are working and to find any drug adverse effects.

- **Imaging studies**: To track involvement in the heart and lungs, such as echocardiograms and high-resolution CT scans.

"Pulmonary function tests" are a way to monitor your lungs' condition.

Outcomes reported by patients: Monitoring symptoms and quality of life regularly.

The patient's reaction and the emergence of new symptoms or problems should inform the iteration of the treatment plan.

A better way to manage scleroderma is to combine pharmaceutical treatments with lifestyle adjustments, physical and occupational therapy, and regular monitoring. This will improve the patient's long-term outcomes and quality of life.

CHAPTER 6

MY JOURNEY THROUGH SCLERODERMA

It is possible to live a good life despite living with scleroderma if you are well-informed and employ efficient management techniques. For all you need to know about scleroderma, here's a detailed guide.

Things I Do Every Day and How I Adjust

Establishing a Regular Schedule

Symptom management and general health can both benefit from the establishment of regular daily routines. Meditation and light yoga are great relaxation practices that can help alleviate tension and anxiety.

Home Modifications

You can improve your quality of life by making your home easier to access. Take into account:

- Adding bathroom grab bars.

- Making use of specialized cooking utensils made for reduced dexterity of the hands.

- Making sure that things that are used often are close at hand to reduce fatigue.

Health and Personal Hygiene

Preventing skin issues is as simple as practicing proper personal hygiene:

- Moisturisers and gentle soaps should not include any fragrances.

- It is important to moisturize your skin.

- To keep your skin from drying out, don't take hot showers.

Helping with Aches and Pains

The medicine

Medication for inflammation and pain management may be prescribed by your doctor.

Insulinomas, nonsteroidal anti-inflammatory drugs (NSAIDs), and corticosteroids are common choices. Do as your doctor says and let them know if you experience any negative effects.

Non-Medical Approaches

To alleviate aches and pains in the muscles and joints, try using a heating pad or a warm compress.

The use of gentle massage techniques can increase blood flow and alleviate pain.

Occupational Therapy: Working with a trained professional in this field can help you develop skills that will make doing everyday activities easier.

Food and Nutrition Advice

Dietary Balance

Symptom management and general health can both benefit from a balanced diet:

Fruits and vegetables are a great source of antioxidants, vitamins, and minerals.

Include lean proteins such as fish, chicken, beans, and nuts in your diet.

- **Whole Grains**: Choose oats, brown rice, and whole wheat bread.

Particular Dietary Requirements

- **Vitamin D and calcium are crucial for healthy bones, particularly when using corticosteroids.

- **Low Sodium**: The ability to control fluid retention and high blood pressure is improved.

- **Stay away from Alcohol and Caffeine**: These substances can make your symptoms worse and ruin your medication.

Staying Moist

If you want to keep your skin healthy and hydrated, drink lots of water.

Physical fitness and regular exercise

Exercise's Crucial Role

Flexibility, strength, and general health can all benefit from regular exercise. As a bonus, it aids with stress management and lifts spirits.

Exercise Categories

If you're stiff or inflexible, try stretching for a little while.

- **Aerobic Exercise**: Cardiovascular health is improved by activities such as walking, swimming, or cycling.

Light weightlifting is a great way to build muscle and stabilize joints as part of a strength training program.

Personalising Your Workout Routine

Consult a physical therapist to create an individualized program of exercises that takes into account your current fitness level and any restrictions you may have.

Strategies for Mental Health and Coping

Mental Health

The mental health of those who live with chronic illnesses can suffer as a result. Proactively attending to emotional well-being is crucial.

Strategies for Coping

Counseling: Talking to a trained mental health professional can help you learn to manage your emotions and overcome difficult situations.

Joining a support group for people with scleroderma is a great way to get both emotional and practical help.

Meditation, deep breathing exercises, and practicing mindfulness are some of the best ways to relax and boost your mood, which in turn can help alleviate anxiety.

Developing a Network of Caretakers

Lovers and Companions,

If you want your loved ones to be there for you when you need them, they need to know about scleroderma, therefore educate them.

Health Care Group

Maintain open communication with all of your medical professionals, including your family doctor, rheumatologist, and specialists.

Local Assets

To get the help and information you need, look into patient advocacy organizations, online support groups, and community services in your area.

Accommodations for the Workplace

Talking to Workplace Supervisors

Bring up your illness with your boss and ask for the adjustments you need, such as more leeway in your schedule or the option to work remotely.

Legal safeguards

Learn about your legal protections under statutes like the Americans with Disabilities Act (ADA), which mandates that businesses offer reasonable accommodations for people with disabilities.

Real-World Modifications

Adjustable seats and keyboards are examples of ergonomic office equipment that can help reduce strain and discomfort.

Scleroderma and Travelling

Looking Forward

To have a pleasant and trouble-free journey, you should plan:

Be sure to bring any prescription drugs and other medical supplies you may need.

Accessibility: Pick lodgings that are easy to get to and have enough space for everyone.

- **Plan Your Trip**: Make sure to factor in additional time to relax and deal with any symptoms that may arise.

While on the road

To avoid becoming dehydrated, it is important to drink enough water.

Remember to Move around: Whether you're in the car or on an airplane, make sure to get up and move around every so often.

Put on loose, comfy clothes to lessen the likelihood of discomfort. - **Dress Comfortably**.

Help with Budgeting and Financial Planning

Medical Costs: A Comprehensive Overview

Be sure you know what your insurance will cover and how much you will have to pay out of cash before undergoing treatment for scleroderma.

Access to Financial Aid

Seek out patient support programs offered by pharmaceutical companies, grants and subsidies from the government, and non-profit organizations.

Set a budget.

Make a plan to keep track of your money so you can pay for things like healthcare and necessities. Talk to a financial advisor if you need help budgeting for the costs associated with a long-term health condition.

Keep Yourself Informed and Well-Educated

#4 Continual Learning

Read up on scleroderma from credible sources regularly, go to seminars, and join webinars to keep yourself informed.

Studies and Human Trials

To gain access to novel medicines and help advance our understanding of the condition, it is important to stay informed about the most recent research and think about taking part in clinical trials.

Interactions with Medical Professionals

Stay in constant contact with your healthcare providers. If anything about your health or therapy is unclear to you, don't be afraid to ask.

You can improve your quality of life and manage scleroderma more efficiently by using these tactics every day. Keep in mind that scleroderma affects everyone differently; thus, it is essential to discover a treatment plan that works for you and make adjustments as necessary.

CHAPTER 6

MY JOURNEY THROUGH SCLERODERMA

It is possible to live a good life despite living with scleroderma if you are well-informed and employ efficient management techniques. For all you need to know about scleroderma, here's a detailed guide.

Things I Do Every Day and How I Adjust

Establishing a Regular Schedule

Symptom management and general health can both benefit from the establishment of regular daily routines. Meditation and light yoga are great relaxation practices that can help alleviate tension and anxiety.

Home Modifications

You can improve your quality of life by making your home easier to access. Take into account:

- Adding bathroom grab bars.

- Making use of specialized cooking utensils made for reduced dexterity of the hands.

- Making sure that things that are used often are close at hand to reduce fatigue.

Health and Personal Hygiene

Preventing skin issues is as simple as practicing proper personal hygiene:

- Moisturisers and gentle soaps should not include any fragrances.

- It is important to moisturize your skin.

- To keep your skin from drying out, don't take hot showers.

Helping with Aches and Pains

The medicine

Medication for inflammation and pain management may be prescribed by your doctor.

Insulinomas, nonsteroidal anti-inflammatory drugs (NSAIDs), and corticosteroids are common choices. Do as your doctor says and let them know if you experience any negative effects.

Non-Medical Approaches

To alleviate aches and pains in the muscles and joints, try using a heating pad or a warm compress.

The use of gentle massage techniques can increase blood flow and alleviate pain.

Occupational Therapy: Working with a trained professional in this field can help you develop skills that will make doing everyday activities easier.

Food and Nutrition Advice

Dietary Balance

Symptom management and general health can both benefit from a balanced diet:

Fruits and vegetables are a great source of antioxidants, vitamins, and minerals.

Include lean proteins such as fish, chicken, beans, and nuts in your diet.

- **Whole Grains**: Choose oats, brown rice, and whole wheat bread.

Particular Dietary Requirements

- **Vitamin D and calcium**are crucial for healthy bones, particularly when using corticosteroids.

- **Low Sodium**: The ability to control fluid retention and high blood pressure is improved.

- **Stay away from Alcohol and Caffeine**: These substances can make your symptoms worse and ruin your medication.

Staying Moist

If you want to keep your skin healthy and hydrated, drink lots of water.

Physical fitness and regular exercise

Exercise's Crucial Role

Flexibility, strength, and general health can all benefit from regular exercise. As a bonus, it aids with stress management and lifts spirits.

Exercise Categories

If you're stiff or inflexible, try stretching for a little while.

- **Aerobic Exercise**: Cardiovascular health is improved by activities such as walking, swimming, or cycling.

Light weightlifting is a great way to build muscle and stabilize joints as part of a strength training program.

Personalising Your Workout Routine

Consult a physical therapist to create an individualized program of exercises that takes into account your current fitness level and any restrictions you may have.

Strategies for Mental Health and Coping

Mental Health

The mental health of those who live with chronic illnesses can suffer as a result. Proactively attending to emotional well-being is crucial.

Strategies for Coping

Counseling: Talking to a trained mental health professional can help you learn to manage your emotions and overcome difficult situations.

Joining a support group for people with scleroderma is a great way to get both emotional and practical help.

Meditation, deep breathing exercises, and practicing mindfulness are some of the best ways to relax and boost your mood, which in turn can help alleviate anxiety.

Developing a Network of Caretakers

Lovers and Companions,

If you want your loved ones to be there for you when you need them, they need to know about scleroderma, therefore educate them.

Health Care Group

Maintain open communication with all of your medical professionals, including your family doctor, rheumatologist, and specialists.

Local Assets

To get the help and information you need, look into patient advocacy organizations, online support groups, and community services in your area.

Accommodations for the Workplace

Talking to Workplace Supervisors

Bring up your illness with your boss and ask for the adjustments you need, such as more leeway in your schedule or the option to work remotely.

Legal safeguards

Learn about your legal protections under statutes like the Americans with Disabilities Act (ADA), which mandates that businesses offer reasonable accommodations for people with disabilities.

Real-World Modifications

Adjustable seats and keyboards are examples of ergonomic office equipment that can help reduce strain and discomfort.

Scleroderma and Travelling

Looking Forward

To have a pleasant and trouble-free journey, you should plan:

Be sure to bring any prescription drugs and other medical supplies you may need.

Accessibility: Pick lodgings that are easy to get to and have enough space for everyone.

- **Plan Your Trip**: Make sure to factor in additional time to relax and deal with any symptoms that may arise.

While on the road

To avoid becoming dehydrated, it is important to drink enough water.

Remember to Move around: Whether you're in the car or on an airplane, make sure to get up and move around every so often.

Put on loose, comfy clothes to lessen the likelihood of discomfort. - **Dress Comfortably**.

Help with Budgeting and Financial Planning

Medical Costs: A Comprehensive Overview

Be sure you know what your insurance will cover and how much you will have to pay out of cash before undergoing treatment for scleroderma.

Access to Financial Aid

Seek out patient support programs offered by pharmaceutical companies, grants and subsidies from the government, and non-profit organizations.

Set a budget.

Make a plan to keep track of your money so you can pay for things like healthcare and necessities. Talk to a financial advisor if you need help budgeting for the costs associated with a long-term health condition.

Keep Yourself Informed and Well-Educated

Continual Learning

Read up on scleroderma from credible sources regularly, go to seminars, and join webinars to keep yourself informed.

Studies and Human Trials

To gain access to novel medicines and help advance our understanding of the condition, it is important to stay informed about the most recent research and think about taking part in clinical trials.

Interactions with Medical Professionals

Stay in constant contact with your healthcare providers. If anything about your health or therapy is unclear to you, don't be afraid to ask.

You can improve your quality of life and manage scleroderma more efficiently by using these tactics every day. Keep in mind that scleroderma affects everyone differently; thus, it is essential to discover a treatment plan that works for you and make adjustments as necessary.

CHAPTER 7

FEMALE-SPECIFIC FACTORS

What Women Should Know About Scleroderma According to the "Essential Guide to Scleroderma"

The chronic connective tissue illness scleroderma can have a profound effect on many parts of a woman's life. If we want to help women effectively, we need to know how it relates to their specific health issues. This article covers all the bases for women who have scleroderma.

Scleroderma with Pregnancy: What to Expect and How to Treat It

Women who suffer from scleroderma face particular difficulties during pregnancy. It takes meticulous preparation and constant observation by a multidisciplinary medical team, but many pregnant women with scleroderma can have healthy babies.

- **Dangers**: Scleroderma raises the odds of problems like preeclampsia, low birth weight, and premature birth. The presence of internal organ involvement, especially in the kidney and lungs, and the kind of scleroderma (limited vs. diffuse), can impact these risks.

Counseling before conception is crucial for management. Pregnancy should not be attempted unless a woman has achieved illness stability. It is critical to have frequent prenatal appointments with an obstetrician and rheumatologist who are knowledgeable about high-risk pregnancies. Some scleroderma medications, such as methotrexate, are not safe to take while pregnant, therefore it may be necessary to make adjustments to your medication regimen.

Scleroderma and Hormonal Shifts

The development and severity of scleroderma can be affected by changes in hormone levels.

Some women find that their symptoms, like joint pain and exhaustion, become worse throughout their menstrual cycle.

- **throughout and after pregnancy**: Hormonal shifts that occur throughout pregnancy have the potential to impact the severity of the disease. Symptoms may worsen or go into remission for some women after giving birth.

The decline in estrogen levels that occurs during menopause can make symptoms like dryness and joint discomfort worse.

The Health of the Gynaecology

A woman's general health greatly depends on her gynecological health if she has scleroderma.

- **Regular Screenings**: Because scleroderma can raise the risk of cancers, it is vital to have regular screenings for cervical and breast cancers in addition to gynecological exams.

- **Vaginal Health**: Because scleroderma affects the skin, it can cause painful dryness and tightness in the vagina, which can lead to infections. You can alleviate these symptoms with the use of moisturizers and lubricants.

Scleroderma while breastfeeding

Although it may be difficult, it is usually possible to breastfeed while dealing with scleroderma.

- **Medication Management**: It is important to see a healthcare professional to clarify if the drugs used to treat scleroderma are safe to be taken while nursing.

- **Physical Difficulty**: Breastfeeding can be uncomfortable for some women due to Raynaud's phenomenon, which affects the nipples. Warm compresses before eating are one helpful strategy.

Menopause and Managing Its Symptoms

Various ways can menopause interact with scleroderma, necessitating individualized approaches to care.

The therapy of scleroderma can be complicated when symptoms such as hot flashes and joint discomfort coincide with one another.

- Hormone replacement therapy (HRT): Hormone replacement therapy (HRT) is a viable option for addressing severe menopausal symptoms, but it is important to take caution when using it because of the hazards involved.

Genetic Counselling and Family Planning

Women living with scleroderma must take additional precautions while developing a family.

There is no direct hereditary link to scleroderma, although a history of autoimmune disorders in the family can raise the risk. **Genetic Counselling** can help with this. Understanding these dangers can be aided by genetic counseling.

Women with scleroderma, particularly those on teratogenic drugs, must adhere to the strictest guidelines for safe and effective contraception.

Effect on Sexual Wellness

Intimacy and sexual health can be greatly affected by scleroderma.

- **Physical Obstacles**: Conditions including dry vaginal skin, painful joints, and tight skin can all make it difficult to engage in sexual activity.

Emotional Impact: Depression and problems with body image can affect a person's desire for and enjoyment of sexual activity. It can be helpful to seek counseling and to communicate openly with partners.

Positive Body Image and Confidence

The outward manifestations of scleroderma can have a significant impact on one's sense of self-worth and body image.

Outward Signs: Changes to the face, digital ulcers, and thickening of the skin can all have an impact on one's sense of self-worth. Women who are experiencing these changes might find support through counseling and support groups.

Self-esteem can be enhanced through the practice of **empowerment**, which entails partaking in activities like exercise and hobbies that increase confidence.

Making Relationships with Other Women

It is really helpful to connect with other women who are dealing with scleroderma.

Joining a support group is a great way to get both emotional and practical help.

- **Online Communities**: Women all around the world may find each other and share resources through online forums and social media groups.

Awareness and Advocacy

Improving care and research funding for scleroderma requires advocacy and increasing awareness of the disease.

- **Self-Advocacy**: Women can take charge of their health and make an active role in decisions regarding their treatment if they take the time to educate themselves about their condition.

- **Raise Public Knowledge**: One way to raise support for scleroderma research and get the public more informed is to take part in awareness campaigns and fundraising activities.

CHAPTER 8

INVESTIGATIONS AND PLANS FOR THE FUTURE

Recent Developments in the Field

Researchers in the field of scleroderma are making great strides in elucidating the disease's pathophysiology, discovering diagnostic biomarkers, and creating new treatments. The immune system's function, fibrosis's molecular and cellular mechanisms, and the disease's hereditary and environmental components are all areas of investigation. To better personalize treatments for each patient, there is a strong push to uncover unique biomarkers that can foretell how a disease will advance and how a patient will react to treatment.

Recent Progress in Genetics

Several genes have been shown to enhance the likelihood of acquiring scleroderma, according to genetic studies. Genetic variations that affect the immune system, causing an aberrant response and fibrosis, have been discovered through studies. New genetic markers and processes implicated in scleroderma have been discovered thanks to advances in genomics, such as whole-genome sequencing. To create focused treatments and individualized treatment programs, it is essential to understand these hereditary factors.

Potentially Revolutionary New Treatment Approaches

Biologics, small compounds, and antifibrotic drugs are among the novel therapy approaches being researched. To control the immune response and decrease inflammation, biologics are developed. One example is monoclonal antibodies that target certain cytokines. Researchers are also looking at small compounds that can block important signaling pathways related to fibrosis. Furthermore, antifibrotic medications work by inhibiting the fibrotic process itself. More effective management of scleroderma may soon be possible with the help of these therapies, which are now in different phases of clinical studies.

Clinical Trials: How to Take Part and What You Can Gain

To create novel treatments or enhance current ones, clinical trials are crucial. By taking part in clinical trials, patients can get their hands on innovative treatments and all-encompassing healthcare. By participating in clinical trials, patients aid in the search for improved treatments and a better understanding of the disease. Extensive monitoring and follow-up are commonplace in trials, guaranteeing that patients receive top-notch treatment. Patients should talk to their doctors about the pros and cons of participating in a clinical trial before making a decision.

Scleroderma and Personalised Medicine

The goal of personalized medicine is to create unique treatment plans for each patient by analyzing their genetic, molecular, and clinical data. Personalized techniques are gaining significance in the treatment of scleroderma. Clinicians can improve the efficacy of treatment decisions by gaining a thorough grasp of each patient's disease and its unique features, such as genetic markers and biomarkers. Additionally, individuals with a higher risk of severe disease can be identified through personalized medicine, which allows for early intervention and better outcomes.

Patient registries play an important role.

Databases that gather information about scleroderma patients are called patient registries. Researchers can learn a lot about illness trends, results, and treatment responses from the data provided by these registries. Registers make it possible to conduct studies on a massive scale, which can reveal patterns that would otherwise go unnoticed in more modest investigations. By drawing attention to both beneficial and harmful treatment options, they aid in the creation of clinical guidelines and ultimately lead to better patient care.

Research on Stem Cells and Their Possibilities

Scleroderma, especially in its most severe forms, may be treatable with the help of stem cell research. Transplanting a patient's stem cells into their immune system (autologous stem cell transplantation) may alleviate symptoms and delay the course of the disease. Research on mesenchymal stem cells is also underway because of their anti-inflammatory and antifibrotic capabilities. Although they are still in the early stages of development, stem cell therapies show great promise for helping patients who have not responded to more traditional forms of treatment.

Joint Academic Investigations

Scleroderma research can only progress with the help of institutions, patient groups, and individual researchers working together. Patients' backgrounds and experiences are better represented in multicenter studies, and results are more broadly applicable when researchers work together across borders. New medicines can be developed more quickly through collaborative efforts since resources and expertise can be pooled. To raise awareness of the disease, provide financial support, and encourage these partnerships, patient advocacy groups are crucial.

Looking Ahead and Feeling Hopeful

Numerous exciting advancements are on the horizon for scleroderma research, which bodes well for the future. More effective and safer treatments, better early detection, and the discovery of novel therapeutic targets are all goals of ongoing research. The use of state-of-the-art technologies like genomics, proteomics, and AI is set to completely transform the way scleroderma is understood and treated. Hopefully, patients will have better results and a higher quality of life as a result of these innovations.

Ways in Which Patients Can Help Advance Science

There are multiple methods by which patients can help advance scleroderma research. People who take part in patient registries and clinical trials contribute crucial data that fuels new scientific discoveries. The patient voice can be amplified, research goals can be influenced, and research programs can gain financing by engaging with patient advocacy organizations. By providing researchers with first-hand accounts, patients can influence studies that aim to solve practical problems and enhance healthcare. The research community can receive additional assistance from education and awareness initiatives that bring attention to the significance of continuing research on a cure for scleroderma.

All things considered, scleroderma research is a vibrant and promising field. We can make great strides in understanding and treating this complicated disease if patients and the community at large stay informed and actively participate in research initiatives.

CHAPTER 9

CHILDREN WITH SCLERODERMA

How to Spot Scleroderma in Kids

Skin and connective tissue thickening and hardening are hallmarks of the uncommon autoimmune disorder known as pediatric scleroderma. Because scleroderma is rare and its symptoms can vary widely, diagnosing it in youngsters can be difficult. The following could be considered early warning signs:

Thickening, tightness, or hardening of the skin; typically begins on the extremities, face, or hands.

- **Raynaud's Phenomenon**: In this disorder, exposure to cold or stress causes the fingers or toes to turn white or blue.

Inflammation of the joints can lead to swelling, which in turn can cause pain and restrict movement.

- **Weakness in Muscles**: It's possible to experience gradual weakening of the muscles, especially in the limbs.

Issues like acid reflux, trouble swallowing, or impaired intestinal motility are examples of **Gastrointestinal Symptoms**.

The key to effective management and treatment, which can potentially slow down the progression of the disease and improve quality of life, is early detection.

Variations in Signs and Development

There are two primary forms of pediatric scleroderma, which manifest differently in adults:

1. **Sclerosing fibrosis of the skin (morphea)**:

- **Signs**: Usually just visible on the surface and in the deeper layers of tissue. Morphoses can be broadly classified into three types: confined, linear, and generalized.

• **Development**: While it usually doesn't impact vital organs, it can lead to major aesthetic and functional problems in regions like the face or joints.

2. I have systemic sclerosis, often known as scleroderma.

The skin, blood arteries, and internal organs (kidneys, heart, lungs) are impacted. In children, it's more common, although it usually has a worse impact.

Serious problems like pulmonary hypertension, renal crisis, or gastrointestinal involvement might develop as the condition progresses.

For youngsters, the course of the disease can be very unpredictable, with both remission and flare-ups possible.

Problems with Diagnosis in Children's Cases

Scleroderma in children presents unique diagnostic challenges:

- **Rarity**: Delays in diagnosis are typical due to the uncommonness of the condition in youngsters.

The symptoms can be similar to those of other pediatric illnesses, such as lupus or juvenile idiopathic arthritis, which is known as **overlap with other conditions**.

Healthcare practitioners and parents may not see scleroderma as a possible diagnosis due to a lack of awareness.

Here are some diagnostic tools:

- **Clinical Examination**: Thorough evaluation of various symptoms, including changes to the skin and involvement of the joints.

Blood tests to detect inflammatory indicators and particular antibodies (such as ANA and anti-Scl-70) are known as **laboratory testing**.

- **Imaging**: magnetic resonance imaging (MRI), ultrasonography (ultrasound), or other imaging modalities to assess the volume of the affected tissue.

A biopsy of the skin or other tissues may be required to establish a definitive diagnosis.

Approaches to Treating Young Patients

The goals of treating scleroderma in children are symptom management, complication prevention, and quality of life improvement. Methods encompass:

- Health supplements:

Methotrexate, mycophenolate mofetil, or cyclophosphamide are examples of immunosuppressants that can lower the activity of the immune system.

- **Corticosteroids**: For the management of inflammation and episodes of flare-ups.

For pulmonary hypertension and Raynaud's phenomenon, **vasodilators** are prescribed.

For specific areas of skin involvement, use **Topical Treatments**.

- Physical therapy: to avoid contractures and keep joints functioning normally.

Occupational therapy can help with adaptive strategies and everyday tasks.

Skin Care: Protective measures and moisturizers for dry skin and ulcer management.

- **Nutritional Support**: Improving digestion and making sure everyone grows and develops normally.

Help for Families and People Who Care for Them

It is crucial to assist families and carers:

- **Education**: Detailing the illness, available treatments, and anticipated results thoroughly and understandably.

- **Counselling**: Helping families deal with the mental and emotional difficulties of caring for a sick kid.

- **Support Groups**: **Meeting Up**: **LinkedIn** with Other Families Dealing With The Same Thing To Get Advice And Stories.

Respite Care: A short break for carers so they can refuel and continue their work.

Reasons to Think About Education

Educational obstacles may be encountered by children with scleroderma:

- **Assistance at School**: Creating and implementing 504 plans or individualized education programs (IEPs) to deal with issues like exhaustion, medical visits, and physical restrictions.

- **Awareness Among Teachers**: Informing educators about the student's health and any possible accommodations they may require.

- Social isolation can be prevented through the use of **peer support**, which entails promoting understanding and inclusion among peers.

The Effects on Children's Minds

Scleroderma can have a major effect on children's mental health:

Depression, anxiety, and poor self-esteem as a result of physical changes and limits constitute emotional distress.

Dealing with scars and other noticeable skin changes is one example of a **Body Image Issue**.

Problems making and keeping friends are examples of **Social Challenges**.

Children need psychological support, such as therapy or counseling, to overcome these obstacles.

Challenges with Development and Growth

Developmental and growth-related effects of scleroderma include:

- **Growth Delay**: Side effects of medications and long-term health conditions might stunt physical development.

• **Delayed Puberty**: Impacts of diseases and hormonal changes might postpone the onset of puberty.

- **Bone Health**: Inflammation and immobility can lead to bone abnormalities or osteoporosis.

To keep these problems under control, it's best to see a pediatric endocrinologist and dietitian regularly.

Moving on to Care for Adults

The transfer to adult care is critical for children with scleroderma as they mature:

Care is gradually transitioned to adult rheumatologists and other specialists as part of the **Planned Transition**.

Helping young adults learn to take charge of their health on their own is the goal of **Self-Management Education**.

Continuity of Care: Making sure that doctors treating children and adults can talk to one another without any hitches.

Constructing a Network of Children with Scleroderma

Better treatment and advocacy can result from a more cohesive community:

Organizations that focus on scleroderma research, raising awareness, and assisting are known as **Patient Advocacy Groups**.

Forums and social media groups where people may share their experiences and advice make up online communities.

Initiatives to promote public awareness about pediatric scleroderma and to raise funding for research are known as **Fundraising and Awareness Campaigns**.

Families dealing with scleroderma can greatly benefit from establishing a system of mutual aid and support for their children.

CHAPTER 10

RESEARCH AND CARE FOR SCLERODERMA IN THE FUTURE

Improvements in Medical Care:

Improvements in symptom control, decreasing disease progression, and increasing patients' quality of life have been the primary goals of scleroderma treatment efforts during the last decade. When it comes to controlling the illness, traditional medicines such as immunosuppressants and anti-inflammatory medications are still crucial. But new therapy approaches have changed the game for scleroderma care, like biological medicines that target particular pathways in the disease's pathophysiology. There is optimism for better outcomes and disease control thanks to these developments.

Methods for Accurate Medical Care

Using patient-specific data like as genetics, immune system composition, and disease subtypes, precision medicine in scleroderma care develops individualized therapy plans. Clinicians can improve the efficacy of personalized medicines by utilizing modern diagnostic methods such as gene expression profiling and biomarker analysis to address underlying illness causes. By not using a cookie-cutter approach, this method not only improves treatment results but also reduces the likelihood of adverse consequences.

Studies on Specific Treatments

Targeted treatments that specifically alter scleroderma-related fibrotic processes and abnormal immune responses are the subject of active investigation. Some examples of these treatments are gene-based interventions aimed at particular biological targets, small molecule inhibitors, and monoclonal antibodies. There are new opportunities to enhance disease management and even achieve remission through clinical studies that study the safety and effectiveness of these possible medicines.

Biomarkers and Tools for Prediction:

Early diagnosis, prognosis, and therapy monitoring in scleroderma are being improved by advances in predictive techniques and biomarker discoveries. Autoantibodies, cytokine profiles, and imaging modalities are biomarkers that show how the disease is progressing, how well it is responding to treatment, and when to expect the next diagnosis. Better decisions and preventative measures against irreparable organ damage are made possible with the integration of these biomarkers into therapeutic practice.

Research Projects Focused on Patients

Research efforts that put patients first seek to comprehend scleroderma patients' actual experiences, preferences, and requirements. Patients are encouraged to take an active role in their care through these programs, which include psychological support interventions, shared decision-making frameworks, and patient-reported outcomes. Holistic care and better treatment adherence are two outcomes of these programs' emphasis on patient, carer, and healthcare professional teamwork.

International Partnerships and Networks

Healthcare organizations, advocacy groups, and worldwide research consortia are working together to speed up the treatment and study of scleroderma. Overcoming geographical constraints and discrepancies in access to experts, these worldwide networks enable knowledge exchange, research standardization, and resource sharing. These efforts are promoting best practices in scleroderma management on a global scale and driving innovation through fostering collaboration.

Technology and Telemedicine's Impact

Care for scleroderma is changing as a result of technological advancements such as telemedicine, wearables, and digital health technologies. Patients in underprivileged regions or with mobility issues can greatly benefit from telemedicine because it allows for remote consultations, monitoring of disease parameters, and prompt interventions. Treatment pathways that use technology improve accessibility, foster continuity of treatment, and give patients more agency over their health management.

Resolving Inequalities in Access to Healthcare:

The inequalities in scleroderma care that exist in diagnosis, therapy, and supportive care are the primary targets of current efforts to eliminate these disparities. Culturally competent healthcare practices, outreach programs aimed at underprivileged populations, and efforts to lower financial barriers to care are all part of this. All patients should have access to fair health outcomes, hence stakeholders are working to increase diversity and inclusion in clinical practice and research.

Research Areas with High Potential

To modify the disease and attain long-term remission, current scleroderma research is investigating new treatment targets, regenerative medicine methods, and immune modulation tactics. Stem cell treatments, tissue engineering, microbiome regulation, and epigenetic alterations are some of the main areas of study. These new directions could revolutionize the treatment of scleroderma and usher in a golden age of individualized, precision medicine in the field of rheumatology.

Fostering Hope for the Future

Research, therapeutic choices, and patient care are constantly improving, which gives optimism for a better future despite the problems faced by scleroderma. We are making great strides towards better outcomes, a higher quality of life, and a cure for scleroderma through our collaborative efforts, innovative technologies, and patient-centered approaches. The scleroderma community has been a driving force for good change and research and care excellence by encouraging optimism, perseverance, and activism.

www.ingramcontent.com/pod-product-compliance
Lightning Source LLC
Chambersburg PA
CBHW061053250726
48653CB00001B/377